THE TYLENOL STRENGTH ACETAMINOPHEN RAPID RELEASE GELS SAFE USE

Dosage, Precautions, Side Effects, and Responsible Use for Pain and Fever Relief

Dr. L.J. Patricia

Copyright © 2025 by **Dr. L.J. Patricia**

All rights reserved. No part of this publication may be reproduced, stored in a retrieval system, or transmitted in any form or by any means—electronic, mechanical, photocopying, recording, or otherwise—without the prior written permission of the publisher, except for brief quotations used in reviews, articles, or scholarly works.

Table of Contents

Introduction.. 4
    Overview of Tylenol Extra Strength Acetaminophen... 4
    Purpose of This Guide.. 6
    Importance of Responsible Medication Use...... 7

Chapter 1: Understanding Tylenol Extra Strength Acetaminophen... 10
    What Is Acetaminophen and How It Works..... 10
    Key Features of Extra Strength Rapid Release Gels... 12
    Common Uses: Pain and Fever Management 13

Chapter 2: Proper Dosage Guidelines.............. 16
    Recommended Dosage for Adults................... 16
    Frequency and Duration of Use....................... 18
    Special Considerations for Seniors and Those with Medical Conditions.................................... 19

Chapter 3: Safety and Precautions................... 22
    Who Should Avoid Tylenol Extra Strength....... 22
    Potential Interactions with Other Medications. 24
    Using Tylenol Safely with Alcohol or Other Substances.. 26

Chapter 4: Understanding Side Effects............ 28
    Common and Mild Side Effects....................... 28

Serious and Rare Adverse Reactions............. 29
Recognizing Signs of Overdose or Liver Damage.. 31

Chapter 5: Safe Use in Special Populations.....34

Tylenol Use During Pregnancy and Breastfeeding... 34
Considerations for People with Liver or Kidney Conditions..36
Pediatric Use: What to Know and Alternatives 37

Chapter 6: Best Practices for Responsible Use... 40

Reading and Understanding Medication Labels.. 40
Storing Tylenol Properly and Avoiding Expired Products.. 42
When to Seek Medical Advice or Switch to Other Treatments...43

Introduction

Overview of Tylenol Extra Strength Acetaminophen

Tylenol Extra Strength Acetaminophen is a popular over-the-counter medicine used to relieve pain and reduce fever. It contains 500 milligrams of acetaminophen per caplet, which is a higher dose than regular Tylenol. This "Extra Strength" version works fast and is especially helpful for headaches, muscle aches, back pain, arthritis, and menstrual cramps. The "Rapid Release Gels" formula is designed to dissolve quickly in the body, so it starts working faster than regular tablets.

Acetaminophen is not an anti-inflammatory drug like ibuprofen. Instead, it works in the brain to block chemicals that cause pain and fever. It's a good choice for people who can't take NSAIDs (nonsteroidal anti-inflammatory drugs) due to stomach issues or other health conditions.

Even though Tylenol is available without a prescription, it's still important to use it properly. Taking too much acetaminophen can seriously harm your liver. This is why understanding the right dose and timing is so important. Tylenol is safe for most people when used as directed, but it can be dangerous if misused. That's why reading the label, following instructions, and knowing your own health needs is key when taking any medication, especially one as commonly used as Tylenol.

Purpose of This Guide

This guide was created to help everyday people understand how to safely and correctly use Tylenol Extra Strength Acetaminophen Rapid Release Gels. Even though this medicine is sold over the counter, that doesn't mean it's risk-free. Many people take pain relievers without fully understanding how they work, how much to take, or when to stop. That's where this guide comes in—to make things clearer and easier for everyone.

We'll explain the basics of what Tylenol does, how to take it the right way, and what to avoid. We'll also look at who should be extra careful when using it, such as people with liver problems or those taking other medications. You'll also learn about side effects, warning signs to watch for, and how to store the medicine safely.

Our goal is to give you trustworthy, easy-to-read information so you can make smart choices. Whether you use Tylenol often or only now and then, knowing the facts can protect your health. With the right knowledge, you can get the relief you need without putting yourself at unnecessary risk. This guide is not a replacement for medical advice, but it is a helpful tool to use along the way.

Importance of Responsible Medication Use

Taking medicine responsibly is one of the most important things you can do for your health. Just because a drug is sold without a prescription doesn't mean it's completely safe to use however you want. Tylenol Extra Strength Acetaminophen is a perfect example. It works well for pain and fever, but taking too much—even by accident—can seriously damage your liver and cause long-term health problems.

Being a responsible medicine user means reading the label carefully every time, even if you've taken it before. You should always double-check the dosage and pay attention to how often you're taking it. If you're using other products that might also contain acetaminophen (like cold or flu medications), it's important not to double up by mistake.

Responsible use also means knowing when to ask a doctor for advice—like if your pain lasts more than a few days, or if you have other medical conditions. Keeping your medicine in a safe place, away from children or anyone who might misuse it, is also part of being careful.

When you take medication responsibly, you protect your health, avoid dangerous side effects, and make sure the medicine can do what it's meant to do: help you feel better safely.

Chapter 1: Understanding Tylenol Extra Strength Acetaminophen

What Is Acetaminophen and How It Works

Acetaminophen is a very common medicine used to relieve pain and reduce fever. You may also hear it called paracetamol in some parts of the world. It doesn't treat the cause of pain or fever, but it helps make you feel better by changing the way your body senses and responds to it.

It works by blocking a substance in the brain called prostaglandins. These substances help carry pain and fever signals through your body. When acetaminophen lowers the amount of prostaglandins, your brain doesn't receive strong signals, and you don't feel as much pain or heat. That's why acetaminophen is often used for headaches, muscle aches, backaches, toothaches, and fevers.

Unlike some other pain relievers like ibuprofen or aspirin, acetaminophen doesn't cause stomach upset or thin your blood. That makes it a safer choice for people with sensitive stomachs or those who can't take other medicines. However, it's important to use the right amount because taking too much can hurt your liver. Overall, acetaminophen is a reliable and gentle option for fast relief when used properly.

Key Features of Extra Strength Rapid Release Gels

Tylenol Extra Strength Rapid Release Gels are a special form of acetaminophen made for fast and powerful relief. Each capsule contains 500 milligrams of acetaminophen, which is a higher dose than regular Tylenol. That means it's designed to relieve stronger pain or bring down a high fever more effectively. But what really makes this product different is how quickly it works.

These gels use a special technology called "rapid release." Inside each capsule are tiny holes or openings that let the medicine get out and into your body faster than traditional tablets. The liquid-gel coating also helps it break down quickly in your stomach. As a result, many people start to feel relief within 15 to 30 minutes.

The capsules are small and easy to swallow, even for people who usually have trouble with pills. They're often used by adults who need fast relief from headaches, cramps, sore muscles, or other kinds of body pain. It's very important to follow the dosing instructions on the label and not take more than needed, especially because of the higher strength. When used correctly, these rapid release gels can offer strong, dependable relief in a short amount of time.

Common Uses: Pain and Fever Management

Tylenol Extra Strength Rapid Release Gels are mainly used for managing pain and reducing fever. People use them for all kinds of everyday pain—headaches, muscle aches, arthritis, toothaches, menstrual cramps, and even minor back pain. These gels are a go-to for many people because they work fast and don't upset the stomach like some other pain medicines can.

They're also great for bringing down a fever. Whether it's a fever from the flu, a cold, or an infection, acetaminophen helps cool the body down. By working directly in the brain to control temperature, it helps you feel more comfortable while your body fights off illness.

Many people keep Tylenol Extra Strength in their medicine cabinet for when pain or fever strikes. It's safe for most adults when taken as directed and doesn't cause drowsiness, so it won't interfere with your daily activities. However, it's not meant for long-term or daily use unless a doctor says it's okay.

These gels are very helpful during colds, after dental work, or following a workout. Just be sure to never go over the daily dose and don't mix it with alcohol or other products containing acetaminophen. When used properly, they offer fast and trusted relief.

Chapter 2: Proper Dosage Guidelines

Recommended Dosage for Adults

For most healthy adults, the typical recommended dose of **Tylenol Extra Strength Acetaminophen Rapid Release Gels** is **two capsules (1,000 mg) every 6 hours**, as needed for pain or fever. Each capsule contains 500 mg of acetaminophen. You should **never take more than 6 capsules (3,000 mg) in 24 hours**, unless your doctor tells you otherwise.

It's really important to read the label and follow the instructions exactly. Just because the medication is over-the-counter doesn't mean it's completely risk-free. Taking too much acetaminophen can **seriously damage your liver**. That's why sticking to the recommended dose is key.

If you're also taking other medications that contain acetaminophen—like cold or flu medicines—**add those amounts up**, too. Many people don't realize how easy it is to go over the safe limit without noticing. When in doubt, ask your pharmacist or doctor.

Also, **don't take more than two capsules at one time**, and don't try to "double up" if you miss a dose. Tylenol works best when used **only when needed**, not on a fixed schedule unless a doctor has advised it.

Always keep a written schedule or set reminders if needed. It helps prevent accidental overuse.

Frequency and Duration of Use

You can take Tylenol Extra Strength Rapid Release Gels **every 6 hours**, but **not more than 4 times a day**. Even if the pain or fever is really bad, it's not safe to take more than the maximum daily amount. If the pain keeps coming back or lasts several days, it's a sign that you may need to see a doctor.

Tylenol is not meant to be taken continuously for long periods unless your healthcare provider has told you it's okay. For **pain**, you should not use it for **more than 10 days in a row**. For **fever**, it should not be used for **more than 3 days** unless a doctor approves it.

Overuse or long-term use can be harmful, especially to your liver. Many people make the mistake of thinking that more medicine will give quicker or stronger relief. But with Tylenol, **more is not better**—it can be dangerous.

If you need to use it daily for chronic pain (like arthritis or back pain), talk to your doctor about safer long-term options or routine liver monitoring. Always take the **lowest dose** for the **shortest amount of time** that gives you relief.

And remember—if the pain doesn't get better, don't just keep taking pills. Get medical advice.

Special Considerations for Seniors and Those with Medical Conditions

Older adults and people with certain health conditions need to be extra careful when using Tylenol Extra Strength. As we age, our bodies break down medicines differently. This means acetaminophen can stay in the system longer and may be more likely to cause side effects—especially liver problems.

If you're a **senior** (typically age 65 and older), it's often safer to **stick with a lower total daily dose**, like 3,000 mg or even less. Some doctors may recommend **2,000 mg per day** depending on your health status. Always check with your healthcare provider before starting or continuing regular use.

If you have **liver disease, chronic alcohol use, or kidney issues**, you should be extremely cautious. Tylenol can be risky in these cases, even at regular doses. People with **heart disease** or **diabetes** should also speak with their doctors first, because some other medications can interact with acetaminophen.

It's also important to avoid drinking **alcohol while using Tylenol**, since both can harm your liver. Even one or two drinks combined with regular doses can be risky.

Always tell your doctor about all the medications and supplements you're taking. This helps avoid dangerous combinations and keeps you safe while getting pain or fever relief.

Chapter 3: Safety and Precautions

Who Should Avoid Tylenol Extra Strength

While Tylenol Extra Strength is safe for many people, there are some who should avoid using it. People with **severe liver problems**, such as liver failure or chronic hepatitis, should not take this medicine. Tylenol contains **acetaminophen**, which is processed by the liver. Taking it when your liver isn't working well can cause serious damage.

If you are **allergic to acetaminophen**, you must avoid this drug completely. Signs of an allergic reaction can include rash, swelling, itching, or trouble breathing. Also, people who **regularly drink a lot of alcohol** (more than three drinks a day) should not take Tylenol Extra Strength without a doctor's advice. Alcohol and acetaminophen together can increase the risk of liver damage.

Those who are already taking other medications that contain acetaminophen need to be very careful. It's easy to take too much without realizing it, and that can be dangerous. If you're pregnant, breastfeeding, or have kidney disease, it's best to check with your doctor before using Tylenol Extra Strength. Always read labels and follow directions closely. When in doubt, talk to a pharmacist or healthcare provider before taking any medication.

Potential Interactions with Other Medications

Tylenol Extra Strength may seem like a simple pain reliever, but it can interact with other medications in ways that may be harmful. One of the biggest concerns is **taking more than one drug that contains acetaminophen**. Many cold, flu, and allergy medicines already have acetaminophen in them. If you take Tylenol along with those, you might accidentally take too much and hurt your liver.

Some **blood thinners** like **warfarin (Coumadin)** can be affected by Tylenol. Taking acetaminophen regularly may increase the risk of bleeding, especially if you're on a high dose or take it for many days in a row. Your doctor may need to check your blood more often if you use both.

Certain **seizure medications** or **tuberculosis drugs** (like isoniazid) may also interact with Tylenol by making your liver work harder. Over time, that can cause liver stress or damage. Also, if you're on medications that affect the liver, combining them with Tylenol might not be safe.

Always check your medication labels. If you're unsure whether something contains acetaminophen or if it's safe to mix, ask your doctor or pharmacist. Never assume it's okay just because it's sold over-the-counter.

Using Tylenol Safely with Alcohol or Other Substances

One of the most important warnings about Tylenol Extra Strength is not to mix it with **alcohol**. Both alcohol and acetaminophen are processed through the **liver**, and using them together increases the risk of serious liver damage. Even moderate drinking—like a couple of beers or glasses of wine—can be dangerous if you also take high doses of Tylenol or take it often.

The danger grows with regular alcohol use. If you drink heavily or daily, you should talk to a doctor before taking Tylenol at all. In fact, doctors often suggest **limiting acetaminophen to a much lower dose or avoiding it entirely** if you drink often.

Other substances can also raise risks. **Illicit drugs**, especially those that affect the liver or the way medications are broken down, can interfere with Tylenol. Even **natural supplements**, like kava or some herbal remedies, can cause liver stress when used with acetaminophen.

To be safe, avoid taking Tylenol if you've been drinking alcohol recently or plan to drink soon. If you're unsure whether a supplement or drug is safe to use with Tylenol, ask a healthcare provider. It's always better to be cautious when it comes to your liver and your health.

Chapter 4: Understanding Side Effects

Common and Mild Side Effects

Tylenol Extra Strength Acetaminophen Rapid Release Gels are generally safe when used the right way. Still, like any medicine, they can cause some mild side effects in certain people. The most common ones are upset stomach, nausea, or a light headache. Some people also report feeling a bit drowsy or dizzy after taking it. These side effects usually go away quickly and don't cause serious problems.

Sometimes, your body just reacts a little differently to a medicine, especially if it's your first time taking it. If you notice things like bloating, mild skin itching, or a strange taste in your mouth, these are not unusual. You can drink water, rest, or eat something light to help ease these effects.

It's important to read the label and not take more than what's recommended. Taking more won't make the pain go away faster—it can actually make you feel worse. If any mild side effect lasts more than a few days or gets annoying, it's smart to talk to your doctor or a pharmacist. They can help figure out if it's okay to continue or if you should try something else that works better for your body.

Serious and Rare Adverse Reactions

Serious or rare side effects from Tylenol Extra Strength are not common, but they can happen—especially if the drug is misused, mixed with alcohol, or taken in large amounts. One of the most dangerous problems is liver damage, which we'll talk more about in the next section. But besides that, there are other serious reactions you should be aware of.

Some people may have an allergic reaction to acetaminophen. Signs of this include swelling of the face, lips, or tongue, trouble breathing, or a rash that spreads quickly. This kind of reaction is a medical emergency, and you should call 911 or go to the hospital right away.

Another rare but serious condition is called Stevens-Johnson Syndrome—a severe skin reaction that can cause painful blisters, peeling skin, and fever. Though it's extremely rare, it's still a reason why it's important to take this medicine carefully and stop if you see signs of a bad reaction.

If you're taking other medications—especially blood thinners or drugs that affect your liver—you should talk to your doctor before using Tylenol Extra Strength. Serious side effects can often be avoided by staying within the safe dose and keeping your healthcare provider informed.

Recognizing Signs of Overdose or Liver Damage

Taking too much Tylenol—even by accident—can seriously hurt your liver. That's why it's very important to know the signs of an overdose or liver damage. Sometimes, people don't feel anything right away after taking too much, but the damage can still be happening inside the body. The first signs can show up within 24 hours.

Early symptoms of an overdose include nausea, vomiting, loss of appetite, and feeling very tired or confused. Some people also feel pain in the upper right side of the stomach, which is where the liver is located. As the liver gets more damaged, your skin or eyes might start turning yellow—a condition called jaundice. That's a big warning sign and means you need emergency help.

Other signs of serious liver problems include dark-colored urine, pale or gray stool, and bleeding easily. If you or someone else may have taken more than the recommended amount—even just a little—it's best to get medical help immediately. Don't wait for symptoms to get worse.

The good news is that liver damage from Tylenol can often be treated if it's caught early.

That's why it's so important to follow dosage directions and never mix Tylenol with alcohol or other medications without checking first.

Chapter 5: Safe Use in Special Populations

Tylenol Use During Pregnancy and Breastfeeding

Many pregnant women worry about what medications are safe to take during pregnancy. Tylenol (acetaminophen) is one of the most commonly recommended pain relievers for pregnant women. Doctors often say it's okay to use Tylenol in small doses when needed, especially for things like headaches, fever, or back pain. However, it's very important to use the lowest dose for the shortest time possible. Even though it's generally considered safe, using too much or taking it too often could still be risky. Some studies suggest that heavy use of acetaminophen during pregnancy might affect the baby's development, but more research is needed.

During breastfeeding, Tylenol is usually safe too. Only a very small amount of the medicine passes into breast milk, and it's unlikely to harm the baby when taken properly. Still, new moms should always check with their doctor before taking any medicine, including Tylenol. Every pregnancy and every baby is different, so it's best to be cautious. When unsure, talk to a doctor or pharmacist, and never mix Tylenol with other medications unless you're told it's okay. The goal is always to stay comfortable and safe while protecting the baby.

Considerations for People with Liver or Kidney Conditions

If you have liver or kidney problems, using Tylenol (acetaminophen) needs to be done with extra care. The liver is the main organ that breaks down Tylenol in your body. If your liver isn't working well, taking regular or high doses of Tylenol can cause serious damage, even if you follow the usual instructions. People with liver disease, hepatitis, or a history of alcohol abuse should only take Tylenol if a doctor says it's safe—and never more than the recommended amount. Too much acetaminophen can lead to liver failure, which can be life-threatening.

For people with kidney disease, the risk is also higher. Although the kidneys aren't the main organ that processes Tylenol, long-term or frequent use may put more strain on them. If you have any kidney problems, it's important to speak with your healthcare provider before using Tylenol, even for minor aches or fever.

In both cases, avoid drinking alcohol while using Tylenol. Alcohol and acetaminophen together can seriously hurt your liver. Always read the label, avoid combination drugs that contain acetaminophen, and talk to your doctor about safer alternatives. A little caution goes a long way in protecting your health.

Pediatric Use: What to Know and Alternatives

Tylenol (acetaminophen) is commonly used for children to relieve pain and reduce fever. It's generally safe when used properly, but the key is **getting the dose right**. Children are not just "small adults"—their bodies handle medicine differently. That's why pediatric Tylenol comes in different forms like liquid, chewable tablets, and suppositories, depending on the child's age and weight. Always check the label for the correct dose based on the child's weight, not just age. Using a kitchen spoon can be risky—use a proper measuring device that comes with the medicine.

Giving too much Tylenol can be dangerous and may damage the child's liver. Accidental overdose is a common reason for emergency room visits, so keep the bottle safely stored out of reach. Never give adult Tylenol to a child unless a doctor approves it.

If you're looking for alternatives, ibuprofen (like Children's Motrin or Advil) can be used in children older than 6 months, but it's not for kids with certain health problems. Also, natural methods like rest, fluids, lukewarm baths, or cool compresses can help with fever and discomfort.

Always call your pediatrician if you're unsure. When it comes to kids, it's better to ask too many questions than too few.

Chapter 6: Best Practices for Responsible Use

Reading and Understanding Medication Labels

Reading a medication label might seem simple, but it's one of the most important steps to using Tylenol Extra Strength Acetaminophen safely. Every bottle has a Drug Facts label, and every section tells you something critical. Start by looking at the **active ingredient**—in this case, **acetaminophen**. This tells you what's inside the medicine that helps relieve pain or reduce fever.

Next, look at the **dosage instructions**. It will say how many pills to take, how often, and the maximum number of pills per day. It's important not to go over that limit, because too much acetaminophen can harm your liver.

Pay attention to the **warnings section**. This tells you when not to take the medicine, what side effects to watch out for, and when to talk to a doctor. There's also a section about **other ingredients** (like dyes or fillers) in case you have allergies.

Lastly, look for information on **storage and expiration**. Don't ignore it—medicine can stop working or even become harmful if not stored correctly. Always read the label each time you take it. Even if you've used it before, manufacturers may update instructions. Taking those few extra seconds can truly protect your health.

Storing Tylenol Properly and Avoiding Expired Products

Proper storage of Tylenol Extra Strength Acetaminophen Rapid Release Gels helps keep the medicine effective and safe to use. The best place to store it is in a cool, dry place—**not** your bathroom. Many people keep medicine in the bathroom cabinet, but the heat and humidity from showers can break down the medication over time. A bedroom drawer or a kitchen cabinet (away from the stove or sink) is a better option.

Always keep the bottle **tightly closed** to avoid moisture or air getting in. Make sure it's out of reach of children and pets. Even if Tylenol seems harmless, it can be dangerous in the wrong hands or if taken in large amounts.

Never use Tylenol past its **expiration date**. Once expired, the medicine might not work the way it should. Over time, the ingredients may break down and become less effective—or even harmful. Check the date on the bottle regularly, and if it's expired, throw it away safely.

Don't flush it down the toilet. Instead, follow local guidelines for disposing of expired medications. Many pharmacies offer take-back programs. Proper storage and disposal are small steps that go a long way in keeping you and your family safe.

When to Seek Medical Advice or Switch to Other Treatments

Tylenol Extra Strength works well for many types of pain and fever, but it's not the right choice for every situation. You should **talk to a**

doctor if you've been using Tylenol for more than a few days and your symptoms haven't improved. It's designed for **short-term relief**, so if your pain or fever keeps coming back, something more serious might be going on.

Also, if you experience any **unusual side effects**—like skin rashes, yellowing of the skin or eyes, dark urine, or stomach pain—stop taking Tylenol and get medical help right away. These could be signs of a liver problem, which is a known risk when acetaminophen is overused or taken incorrectly.

If you have a **medical condition** like liver disease, are taking other medications, or drink alcohol regularly, it's best to talk to your healthcare provider before taking Tylenol at all. They might recommend a different pain reliever that's safer for your situation.

Sometimes, pain is better treated with other methods like **physical therapy**, lifestyle changes, or prescription medications. Your doctor can help you figure out the best plan. Listening to your body and knowing when to ask for help is a smart and responsible part of using any medicine.

Printed in Dunstable, United Kingdom